2am Pg

The Highs and Lows of an Unexpected Diagnosis

Tyrece and Taria Butler

We dedicate this book to Arlene Butler, one of our biggest supporters through this journey. You are and will truly be missed!

November 1, 1951~October 1, 2019

Psalms   121: 1-3
"I will lift up my eyes to the hills—From whence comes my help? My help comes from the Lord, Who made heaven and earth. He will not allow your foot to be moved; He who keeps you will not slumber."

TABLE OF CONTENTS

ACKNOWLEDGMENTS

We are so thankful for every person who is a part of our village, too many to name, but you know who you are. From the beginning, diagnosis day, to present, each and every one of you have been our listening ears, shoulders to cry on, and someone to vent to. You have not only supported us, but you have also supported our desire to help other families. For all these things, we are grateful and blessed to have you in our lives.

INTRODUCTION

As parents or someone preparing for parenthood, we prepare for and expect to deal with the ailments like the common cold, vomiting, scraping of the knee, or broken bones, to name a few. Whether it is your first child or your fifth, nothing can prepare you for your child being diagnosed with a chronic illness and the unknown that comes along with an unexpected diagnosis.

Whether you are a parent, a sibling, a child, a spouse or a friend, becoming a caregiver is a role that many of us did not choose. Yet, we find ourselves taking care of someone who we love without a playbook or a guidebook to help us along the journey. Like many of you, when we first became caregivers, we yearned for something that would help us to understand our new roles.

From Type 1 diabetes to Cancer, Autism to Sickle Cell, Epilepsy to Asthma amongst many other chronic illnesses, your faith will be tested, your parenting will be tested, your relationships will be tested—you will be tested. Yet, through those tests and tribulations, you will find reassurance in knowing that you are not alone. Other parents have been in your shoes. We have been in your shoes and that is what this book is about—providing real, sometimes raw discussions about parenting and caregiving after diagnosis.

We will offer you a glimpse into our lives through both of our eyes. At times, you will hear from me and at times, you will hear from my husband. Collectively, we hope that our story will bring you hope, reassurance, and comfort in knowing that you can still have an abundant and amazing life while dealing with the highs and lows of caring for a child or loved one with a chronic illness.

As this book journeys through our lives since Trace was diagnosed almost four years ago, you will be invited to think, reflect and even process your role as a caregiver. We've had to learn and are still learning how to rework our lives, our family and our relationships in order to manage his diabetes and keep him alive, daily.

2am Parenting is intended to share with you the highs and lows that we have experienced. From dealing with unexpected feelings and emotions to rethinking relationships, this book is grounded in hope. The hope that you, through our story, will be inspired and will be encouraged no matter what you are enduring. Most importantly, we hope that you will walk away knowing that you are not alone.

We stand firmly on our faith knowing that there is power is sharing our story—a story that we hope will bless you on your journey.

Pause & Ponder

Brain dump any thought, feeling or emotion that you have about the diagnosis of your child or loved one...get it all out!

_____

_____

_____

_____

_____

_____

_____

_____

_____

_____

_____

_____

_____

_____

_____

_____

_____

_____

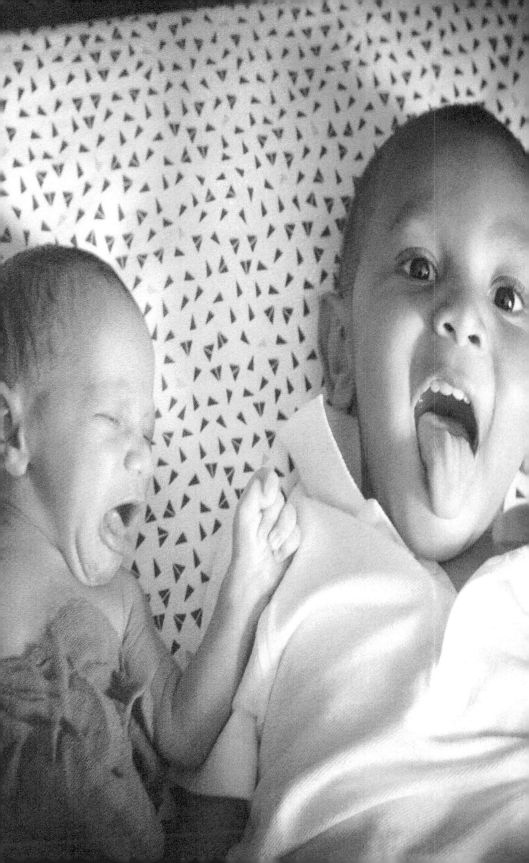

Life Before Diagnosis

"For I know the plans that I have for you, says The Lord."
Jeremiah 29:11

Taria

Tyrece and I met in middle school. We married in the fall of 2010. We enjoyed the typical married life of a young couple. In 2012, we were blessed with our first child, Tate. Shortly thereafter, we had our second son, Trace.

We weren't the Brady Bunch or the Huxtables, but we were your quintessential American family—mom and dad and two loving kids. No, we didn't have the white picket fence, but life was good. At the time, I was a stay-at-home-mom (SAHM), money was tight but nothing like what was to come. We had recently bought a new, bigger, family of four house. Our boys were growing and flourishing. While I stayed at home, Tyrece worked as an Account Manager/Sales Representative for an insurance company. During the week, he traveled for work, which was one of our primary reasons for me to stay-at-home. On weekends, we made sure to make the most of our time—spending time as a family and also time as a married couple.

Early in our oldest son Tate's life, we discovered he could possibly have asthma. At his one-month appointment, his pediatrician heard wheezing in his chest and prescribed breathing treatments. We continued with the breathing treatments throughout his first year of life and at the age of 1 ½ he was hospitalized because of an asthma attack. During the first year of Tate's life, we also discovered what would later be diagnosed as food allergies (all dairy and egg). Managing his asthma and food allergies were our biggest worry or concern at the time and we thought that was difficult. I remember my sister and I were in Target shopping, as many of us love to do; she had a milkshake and Tate begged her for a sip of it. Tate couldn't have been more than 8 months old. My sister, being the aunt that she is, gave in to his "begging" and before we knew it, he was gulping down what was left of the milkshake. Unfortunately for us, no more than 10 minutes later, he was vomiting in the frozen food aisle.

For the most part, in terms of parenting, Tate's allergies and asthma were all that we had to worry about. Tyrece and I were your typical married couple still navigating being the parents of two very young children while also still learning about each other within the scope of our six-year marriage. I can even recall in early January 2016, sending Tyrece the following text message:

I don't want to go into another year of marriage like this......I have 4-5 (caregiver, cook, cleaning and family budgeter/accountant etc.) jobs and I'm exhausted, I need some balance....I am exhausted every day, just my thoughts exhaust me....I feel like a single mother sometimes....not because of you but because I've just continued to operate the way I know how, the way I had to when I was single, I take charge and

figure things out on my own....I don't want to do that
anymore....communication....need to communicate more and better but I need your
help, I don't know how to be vulnerable....I don't know why, I want to be more
relaxed and have more fun in our family and our marriage, I feel so uptight and
anxious all the time....I'm tired!!!

Wow!!! Looking back at the message and tone of that text, I am just speechless! Little did I know that the very things I wanted to change about myself and my marriage were about to be pushed to the limits and tested in a way that I never could have imagined.

Trace was born a perfectly healthy baby boy. Trace was smiling, attempting to hold his head up and stand at one month old. He was always such a chill baby, until he was hungry. Although he didn't mind other people being around, he always seemed to prefer being held by me. Trace also loved trying to keep up with his older brother, eyeing all of Tate's toys as if he couldn't wait to get his hands on them. He was also a much better sleeper than his brother, still not the best, but early on, we could tell he enjoyed his sleep. I would always joke that Trace was a child after my own heart, that he would be the one I could watch a movie with and lounge around with while his brother Tate would be jumping off the bed.

He and his brother got along well. Once we moved into our new home, we made sure to dedicate one bedroom as a playroom for the kids. We could put the boys in there and they would play for hours. Tyrece and I would also sit in the playroom with the boys and play with their cars or football figures with them. Football was and is another huge part of our lives. Tyrece played football at, and graduated from, The University of Michigan. Tyrece and the boys would watch football every Saturday during football season. I can even remember a time that the four of us took a road trip to the "The Big House," The University of Michigan's football stadium. Tate was so excited to be there and to see it for the first time. Tyrece was also excited to show his two boys where he went to college, where he had the opportunity to play football and most importantly, where he made so many lifelong friendships.

12

Despite all appearances of normalcy, throughout the latter part of 2015, Trace began to soak through his diapers and started to exhibit extreme

thirst, which we attributed to teething. The increase in diaper changes was attributed to the increased drinking. I discussed the changes with his pediatrician; she believed he was demanding more milk because we were giving into his demands and assured me he would be fine once we began to cut back on what we allowed him to drink.

Yet, on January 19, 2016, our lives changed forever. I noticed that Trace became very lethargic and could barely move or hold his head up to drink from a cup but he was crying for and demanding something to drink. Something wasn't quite right. My instinct as a mother told me so.

The worse fear that any parent could have, became our reality—our baby was very sick. Our 18-month-old was diagnosed with Type 1 diabetes (Type 1). After taking him to his pediatrician's office, we were told to take him to the ER immediately. Trace had a blood sugar of 1,000 (his normal goal range is 100-200) and he could have lost his life had we waited any longer.

During this time, I felt every emotion possible and in full disclosure, I was angry, overwhelmed, anxious and sad. And in full transparency, I still experience this range of emotions often. I don't understand why God has placed this on us but we're trusting Him and His plan for our family and for Trace's life.

We trust that God will allow us to learn all that we can about managing this disease, that God will help us parent Trace while managing this disease and we pray that God will use this diagnosis to make Trace a stronger child and person. We have a long journey ahead of us and there are good days and not so good days but....In all things, give Him praise!

I remember the first night in the hospital with Trace, I was up somewhere between 2a-3a, holding him because he couldn't sleep, he had been crying a lot through the night. Trace didn't understand what was going on, why we weren't home, why he couldn't have a cup of milk as he normally would. There was a PICU nurse (sent by God) that previously told me she too had a son with Type 1 and that she personally knew what we were going through.

I asked if she was still on duty, I wanted to ask her some questions.

As I sat in the hospital room on the uncomfortable blue couch, I asked her several questions. My first question was what would Trace's daily schedule and routine be now and how it would change. At this time, Trace was still your average toddler, exploring what foods he did and didn't like. Would we have to begin limiting what he did or didn't eat? Secondly, would Trace be limited by this diagnosis?

Would he still be able to be an active little boy, would he still be able to play and rough house with his brother? Lastly, my most pressing question that no doctor or nurse not living the Type 1 life could answer was how would the diagnosis (really) change our lives. At the time, I didn't know I was already experiencing one of the biggest changes.....being awake in the wee hours of the morning, holding him, caring for him, praying for him, checking his blood sugar or just checking on him to make sure he was still breathing.

Ironically, I was pregnant with Trace when our oldest son, Tate, was admitted in the hospital for an asthma attack, now almost exactly two years later, we found ourselves back at the same hospital for Trace.

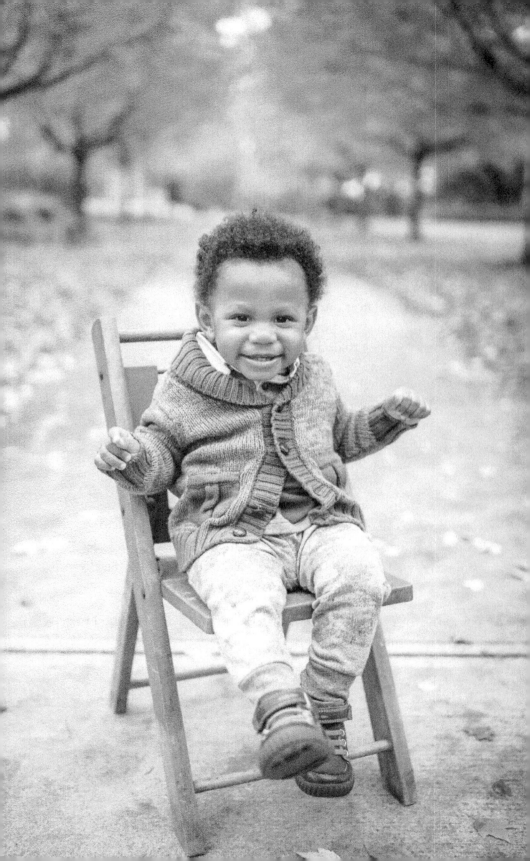

Tyrece

It was a typical Tuesday morning. I was at work joking around with my coworkers when I received a text from my wife, Taria, but the text wasn't really a text, it was a picture. I vividly recall a picture of Trace, laying on the floor, looking as if he was in a daze. Before I could even begin to respond to her text, Taria called me.

"Hey, did you get my text of the picture I sent?"

"Yea, I was just about to respond, what's going on?"

I paused as I could hear the angst in her voice as she began to explain, "Trace is really lethargic, he can barely keep his head up and constantly asking for something to drink."

She went on to tell me that she was going to call the pediatrician because something just didn't seem right. I waited for what seemed like hours. In reality, it was probably no more than 10 minutes before she called back. After speaking with the nurse at the pediatrician's office, Taria said "I am taking him to the pediatrician. After telling the nurse Trace's symptoms, she said I can bring him in now or wait until tomorrow, I can't wait until tomorrow to see what's wrong with him. I will give you a call once we get there and I've talked to the doctor. Keep your phone near you!" I asked if I should leave work and meet them there but Taria said they may be done at the doctor's office by the time I was able to get there from my office.

As soon as the call ended, I immediately started praying, "Please Lord don't let it be something serious ".

I was hoping that at the worst, it was the flu or a bad case of dehydration. I tried to resume what I was working on, but I couldn't. All I could think about was my baby boy as I sat at my desk. I was extremely nervous and could not focus on work. I was trying to be calm and not let my coworkers see me uneasy. After the longest 45 minutes of my life, Taria called me back, frantically crying. All I heard was "meet us at the ER, Trace has diabetes".

Although I heard everything that she said and could fully digest it intellectually, I didn't fully understand what this meant but I knew this was not good at all. I told my coworker there was a family emergency and I had to leave right now. When I got into my car, I screamed as loudly as I could with no care as to who could hear me. I also began to cry. As I was driving to the ER, all I kept saying was, "Please don't take my baby Lord!"

The drive from my office was about 30 minutes, yet, I don't remember stoplights, getting on the highway or even other cars in route. What I do recall is the range of emotions that I was feeling. I was scared, nervous, and not sure what Trace having diabetes actually meant.

When I got to the ER and saw Trace's small body lying in the large hospital bed, my heart dropped. He was alert but still somewhat out of it and nervous with all the nurses and doctors around him. I held his little hand to let him know it was ok but deep down I was crying and screaming inside. I could not let him see his dad shaken because I am supposed to be his rock.

I listened attentively as the doctor was explaining to Taria and I that Trace was in DKA (diabetic ketoacidosis) and his blood sugar was over 1000. The doctor explained that they were going to have to get a lot of insulin in his body to bring his blood sugar down as quickly and safely as possible. I asked the doctor what does all of this mean? He explained that Trace has Type 1 diabetes and he will depend on insulin for the rest of his life.

After a crazy, whirlwind day and night of constant insulin doses, blood sugar checks, and an accidental overdose of insulin by one of the nurses, the nurses and doctors were finally able to get Trace's blood sugar down. Then the crash course of diabetes management began and we had to learn how to take care of him from this point on.

It was as if we were learning how to care for a newborn baby again. We met with an Endocrinologist, other doctors, nurses, a dietician and a social worker. Taria asked that I bring one of her notebooks from home and she went right into mommy/caregiver mode. I remember her writing down the names of everyone that we met with and every bit of information they shared with us to ensure we didn't forget anything.

This was all really mind boggling and so much to absorb. Just hours earlier, we were enjoying our version of the American dream and now, we were told that our child suffered from a chronic illness of which there was no cure. It would change everything about our family, our dynamic and who we are as parents and a married couple.

The entire experience was stressful, at best. We had to remember to check his blood sugar before he ate or drank anything, remember how to calculate the carbs of what he was going to eat or drink and learn to wrestle with a toddler to give him an injection, several times per day. I immediately felt stressed! We had moments of overwhelming uncertainty as we were told we had to learn these things before Trace could be released.

Through each step of our crash course, we experienced a wide range of emotions. Everything was still raw so we were extremely sad, confused and wondering why our son had to go through this. We have an 18-month old child and we have to monitor his blood sugar and what foods he eats! Why can't this be simple!? Why couldn't we return to our relatively simple lives? We had questions, but not that many answers.

And just like that, anyone's life can change and one's faith can be shaken.

Even as Christians, so many feelings and emotions can run through your body. One big one is guilt: "Did I, or we, cause this?" Taria started thinking about caving to her cravings and drinking Pepsi a few times while we were pregnant. Trace was 18 months old when he was diagnosed, he breastfed for about 8 months and at this point in his life, he had never had any candy—a treat for him were Gerber puffs. He was still ex experimenting with some foods; yet, his course selection consisted of nuggets or turkey hot dogs and green beans or peas. I still couldn't help wondering what I or we did wrong! Yes, guilt and even some blaming began to seep in; yet, through it all, I knew that as husband and father, I had to be strong for my family and an assurance to them that we would get through this and be ok. And although I had a greater sense of duty to help more and take on more of the responsibilities as caregiver for Trace, it took some time for me to fully accept this as my new reality.

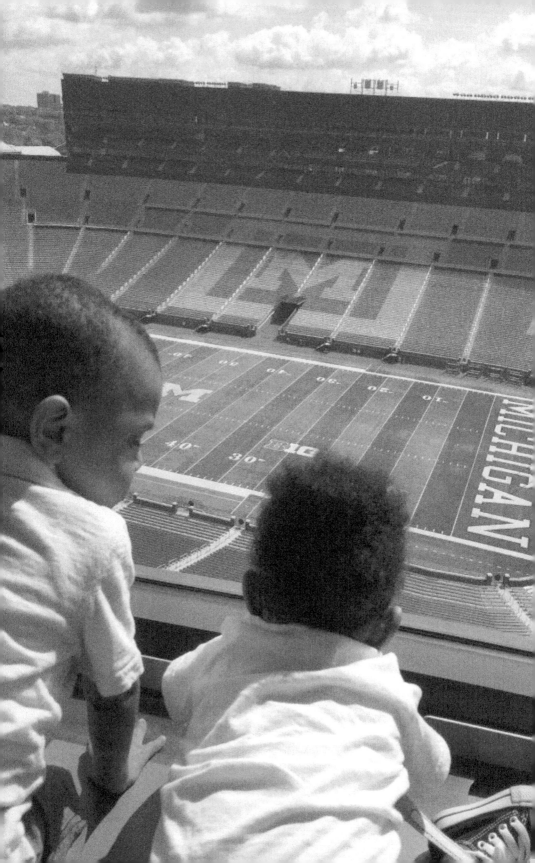

What was life like for you before diagnosis?

_____

_____

_____

_____

_____

_____

_____

_____

What changes have you made as a caregiver?

_____

_____

_____

_____

_____

_____

_____

_____

Stressed

Anxious

Fearful

Worried

Weak

Laughing

to keep from

crying

Scared

Angry

Tense

Tired

Fear and Anxiety

"Whenever I am afraid, I will trust in You." Psalms 56

Taria

I would never consider myself a fearful or anxious person. I've had fearful or anxious moments like the uncertainty of a job interview or when I learned my home had been broken into before I was married, those types of fear and uncertainty. I've never been in or experienced a constant state of fear until I had kids. The fears I've had once I had my kids are fear of harm or danger coming to my children, fear that they will be treated unfairly in this cruel world, or the fear of how my parenting decisions will impact their future selves. Since Trace was diagnosed, I find myself fearful or anxious of many situations and experiences. I am fearful of death, I am fearful of not having his supplies on us when we leave the house, I am fearful of what the constant low and high blood sugars will do to his body and cognitive abilities. Fear creeps in when I wake up from a night of uninterrupted sleep, the first day of school, the first time at summer camp, going on vacation with the kids, going away for a night without the kids...the list

23

could go on and on. I am constantly thinking about the "what ifs" ....what if his blood sugar goes really low and I'm not able to get to him or no one at the school notices before it's too late.

When Trace was first diagnosed, I would be the one to get up at night to check his blood sugar. 2am is the designated time given to us by the doctors and nurses at the hospital. I would make sure my alarm was set every night from 1:45am to 2:15am. There were times when I wouldn't hear any of the alarms or I would wake up late. The fear I felt when I would walk in his room is unexplainable. I would fear that he'd had a low or high blood sugar that cause him to be unresponsive or dead. And every time, after putting my hand on his chest to make sure he was breathing and then checking his blood sugar to make sure he was ok, I would silently cry out of relief, cry out of sadness and cry out of anger at myself. And still, to this day, this fear is ever present even with the technology that we now have. Trace has a continuous glucose monitor (CGM) that monitors his blood sugar, day and night, and alerts us of low and high blood sugar readings. We are still up at night, due to the constant beeps and alerts or when technology just isn't working as it should. The monitor is a blessing but also a source of fear and anxiety.

After Trace was diagnosed, we decided I would go back to work and find a position in my field. The level of fear and anxiety I experienced around this entire situation was like no other. First, it was finding a daycare provider that was confident enough to take him, then train the staff on his care, administering insulin, what to do when his blood sugar goes too low or too high. We were blessed that after hearing about my uneasiness about sending him to daycare, my mother-in-law decided she could keep Trace three days per week and we would only have to send him to daycare the other two days. This was a huge sigh of relief. But even during those two days per week, I was praying constantly throughout the day, asking The Lord for him to be ok and for the staff to remember what to do in any situation. I can recall the night before he was to attend daycare for the first time, I was packing up a small bin of snack items, labeled with the carb count for each item and I just burst into tears. Tyrece came in the pantry where I was with a puzzled look on his face and I had no words other than "this is hard, this is one of those small reminders of what we're dealing with."

I experienced my first full-fledged anxiety attack when one night, we didn't have a sensor for his CGM. Something in me took over my mind and it went to a very dark place; I KNEW that was going to be the night I lost my son because I didn't have the technology to alert us if his blood sugar went too low or too high. The anxiety and fear of losing a child is like nothing else that I can imagine. In full disclosure, the feeling of being anxious, overwhelmed and sad come often but I continue to tell myself that God is able, able to keep me, my mind and my son. When I am faced with these anxieties and fears, breathing, praying and reciting the promises of God are what help me make through each anxiety episode. After this first, or at least, most obvious anxiety attack I decided to go to therapy. I had toyed around with the idea of seeing a therapist for a while because I was having a hard time dealing with and accepting Trace's diagnosis. The anxiety attack pushed me to finally follow through with it.

Who says you can't have Jesus and a therapist?!!

Speaking of a therapist, it is perfectly OK if during your journey, you need to reach out to someone. Licensed therapists are valuable resources who can help you unpack your feelings and process what you are experiencing. If you're not comfortable with the idea of seeing a therapist, start with a pastor or clergy person, they can also be valuable resources.

Tyrece

When I think of fear, I think about an old idea as a kid; shaking in your bones, not being brave, not having the courage to stand up to what you're up against. Now, as an adult, father and married man, fear is not being able to do something, to handle something, to not being able to control what is going on around me. Fear takes on an entirely different

25

shape as you get and gain more responsibilities.

Trace was playing basketball at the YMCA in their 4-5 year-old league. Usually with this age group, the children are wandering around or waving at their parents during the game. This one particular game there was a lot of running up and down the court going on. Both teams decided to play hard! I could hear my sons CGM alarm going off. I immediately grabbed an apple juice and ran on the court in the middle of the kid's basketball game. All of the parents at the game thought I was crazy; I could tell by the looks on their faces. I know they were wondering why this 6'3 guy was on the court with an apple juice. This guy's kid can't be that thirsty that it warrants him to dramatically run on the court!

That's what I imagined was going through the minds of some of the parents. Trace even seemed shocked to see me on the court too! He asked me "what's wrong daddy?" I replied, you're going low Trace, a phrase he has gotten so used to hearing. As I made my way back to my seat, I noticed more of the crowd's look on their faces. I realize that most, if not all, of the parents in the crowd had no clue that Trace has Type 1 diabetes but even those that do know don't realize the stress and fears of this disease. But the fear of his possibly passing out in the middle of the gym floor runs through my mind often. Many parents have comfort in watching their children play sports and not have to worry about their child's blood sugar being too low or too high.

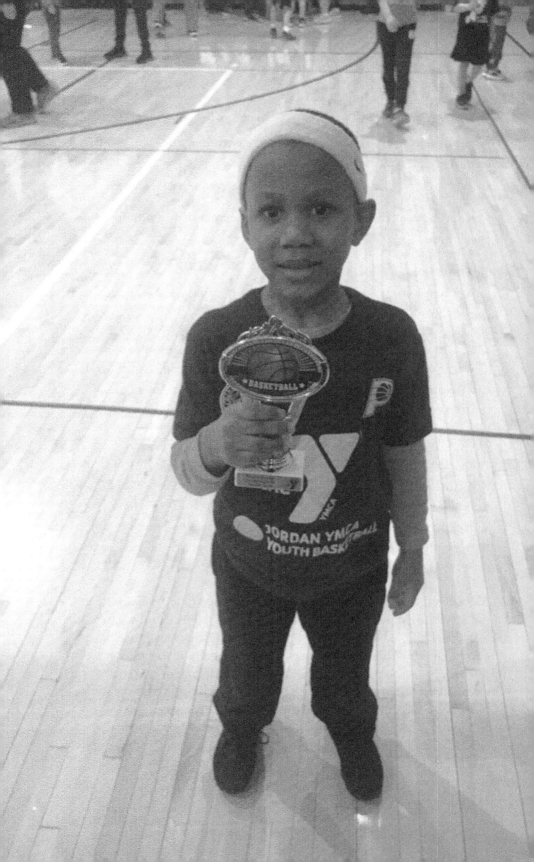

There are so many other fears that come along with managing Trace's chronic illness.......

.......The fear of knowing I may have messed up giving him the wrong insulin dosage.

.......Or the fear that I may not hear my 2am alarm and not get up to check him.

.......When I am traveling for work, I fear that my wife won't get up at 2am to check him.

The fear of watching his blood sugar going up or going down on the CGM app and not being able to reach my wife or whomever is responsible for his care at that moment to let them know to check on him.

And one of my biggest and most intense fears is that I will not be able to afford insulin for my son. I hear the horror stories of families having to ration out insulin because they can't afford it for their child. Through our non-profit organization, we have helped families that had to make the decision on whether to pay for groceries, bills or pay for their child's insulin.

Along with this fear, is also the fear that my insurance will decide to not cover the necessary supplies to take care of Trace and his needs. I fear that I will have to take a job I don't like just because they have good benefits. These past few years, the company I worked for was in the process of being purchased. Along with the talk of whether or not we would retain our positions, there was also talk of a new insurance plan. Some people in my company were saying that the plan was great and some were saying the plan was going to be awful. So many emotions and fears kicked in! How am I going to pay for the supplies needed to keep my son alive! Lord please help me!

Proverbs 3:5 Trust in the Lord with all your heart; and lean not to your own understanding.

I never thought I would experience anxiety. I have experienced anxiety every day since Trace's diagnosis. There are so many scenarios that trigger my anxiety like the alarms on Trace's CGM, him playing outside for long periods or going to restaurants and not knowing the food carb count in order to give the correct amount of insulin.

It's like every day is crunch time and life is on the line. Sometimes I feel like there is no time to relax and take a deep breath.

One evening, Tate expressed to me that he wished I spent more time with him like I do Trace.

I said, "Tate, I do spend a lot of time with you."

His response was "but you're always worried about him" as his face frowned.

Then I realized it wasn't about time, he felt like I was being more attentive toward Trace than I was toward him. I explained to Tate that I need to make sure that Trace is ok and I am still trying to get a handle on this illness. I also told him that I loved him and there are no favorites. As a parent of two boys, I fear that Tate will have resentment towards us or Trace because of Trace's illness and hold a grudge against him. As such, I try to spend quality, one-on-one time with both of my boys so they get dad's full attention and love.

This also happens with couples as one parent seems to be so absorbed in a child or parent's diagnosis that they forget their spouse. My wife and I try to make date nights a must! We know it is crucial that couples spend quality time together. It's like every day is crunch time and life is on the line. Sometimes I feel like there is no time to relax and take a deep breath.

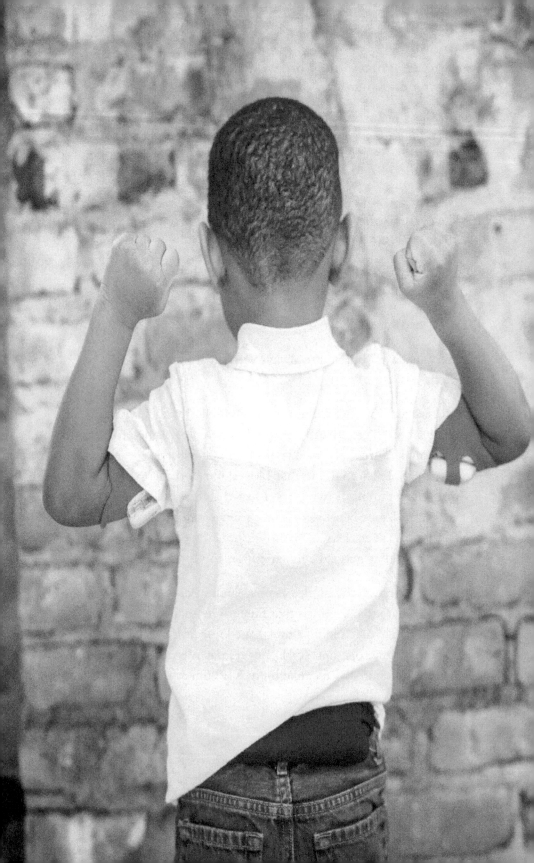

Identify 5 new fears as a caregiver:

_____

_____

_____

_____

_____

What are your fear triggers?

_____

_____

_____

Has fear or anxiety caused you to change or alter anything in your life?

_____

_____

_____

If so, how or what?

_____

_____

_____

How do you combat your anxiety?

_____

_____

_____

GOD IS SOVEREIGN OVER EVERYTHING,
BE GUIDED BY THANKFULNESS
AND TRUST NOT FEAR.

"INTERRUPT ANXIETY WITH GRATITUDE AND PRAISE"

~ANONYMOUS~

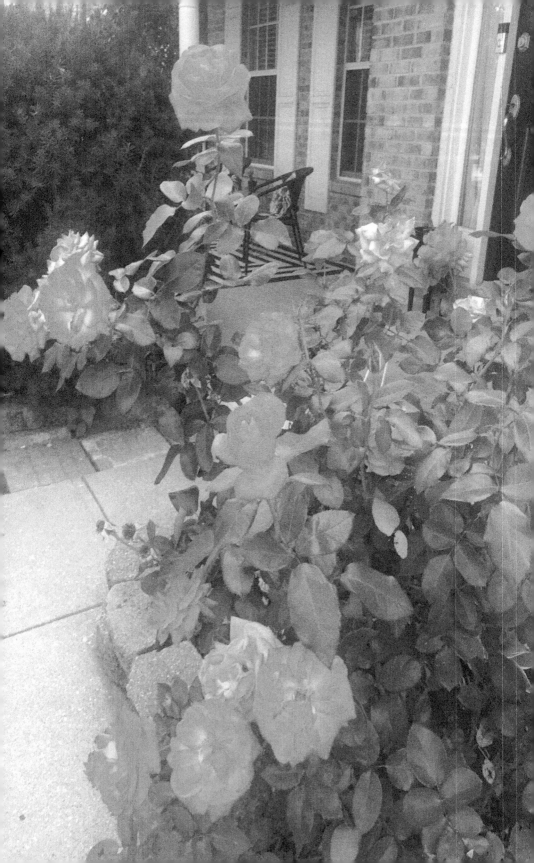

Grief

"...do not sorrow, for the joy of the Lord is your strength"
Nehemiah 8:10

Taria

Grief is.......

Heartbreaking, powerful, gut wrenching, leaves you speechless at times, can also bring peace, calmness and can strengthen your faith. It is something that we all experience at times in our lives and it's HARD, no matter who you are. As a school counselor, I've learned about grief counseling and the stages or cycles of grief. As a person, I've experienced grief and loss of loved ones in my life. But neither of these facets of my life helps or eases the constant grief I experience as we navigate life with a chronically ill child.

It's funny that as we plan or daydream about our lives, we never consider the things that could go wrong. Tyrece and I planned and talked about what schools our kids would attend and what sports or other activities they would possibly participate in. We have a bucket list of places to visit as a family and for just the two of us. So many plans and possibilities had been discussed before Trace was diagnosed. Can we still accomplish these things? Absolutely! But it won't be as easy as once expected. Our "new normal" was not what I had envisioned or what I had dreamt of. And because of this, I've had a hard time "coming to grips" with this "new normal". It is especially hard when you're dealing with a chronic illness that can change from day-to-day. One day, you may feel as if you have a good grasp on things, almost feeling like an expert, and the next day can knock you off your feet and bring you back to square one.

Because of the grief I experience, I decided to try therapy because the grief and anxiety were getting the best of me and I couldn't understand why. I'm a counselor, I'm a Christian, I understand grief. Why am I still grieving? When will I fully accept this life? With every new circumstance or experience, I grieve the "normal" life I thought we'd have and my child would have. My therapist explained to me that this type of grief is different, it's like experiencing the initial shock of a death over and over again with each new experience. This isn't what I thought my life as a parent would be! I envisioned us dropping our kids off to grandma's house on a Friday night for date night or play dates with friends and their kids without worry. I also wanted to just drop them off at summer camp or at school on the first day without having to be sure that everyone knows Trace has Type 1 diabetes, how to take care for him, the signs of low and high blood sugar and how to administer his insulin.

Going to see a therapist, along with my continual praying and relationship with God, brought me some relief, it was like a light-bulb moment: It's okay to continue to grieve. It's okay to experience grief one moment and have peace and joy in the next. I have not "arrived" in dealing with or experiencing grief, and that's ok, I lean on my faith and know my faith will get me through.

"You can mourn and have peace and joy at the same time."

Tyrece

Society has taught us that grief only takes place when you lose someone. Truth is, you can grieve many things. I didn't realize that I was experiencing grief without losing a loved one in my caregiving journey. I thought I was just feeling frustrated or a little saddened but I didn't have a name for what I was experiencing. It wasn't until I talked to my wife about how I was feeling that she told me that I was grieving. I was shocked but it made sense. I didn't lose a loved one, but I was losing certain experiences.

As a caregiver, people don't realize the time you put in to take care of a person. They also don't realize the precious time that you lose. Time is very important in anyone's life. We only have a certain amount of time on this earth, but we don't know how much time that will be. I find myself sometimes wondering, where did the time go in a 24-hour day. It is not uncommon for a caregiver to grieve their time and not know that they are grieving. Along with grieving time, you may also find yourself grieving friendships or other relationships.

Grieving friendships is very common in a caregiver's journey. These friendships are vital to our well-being. Being able to share a bond with a person helps us mentally and emotionally. Sometimes as a caregiver we can lose those relationships because we are so devoted to our mission to take care of our loved one that needs our help. We often forget that maintaining those relationships is important in keeping us connected with our friends and family. It's good to hear and see something different than the same old monotony that we as caregivers experience. We must make it a priority to maintain those relationships. Sometimes when we unconsciously shut out friends and family, we become angry because we expect them to read our minds or automatically know what we're dealing with. I have to remember communication goes both ways.

However, grief is not just about shifting relationships with people, there are other things that may change or dissolve in the life of a caregiver. As I will discuss in greater detail in the next chapter, financial grief can be and is stressful when taking care of a loved one. Let's face it, we cannot survive without money. This kind of grief can cause major health problems. The visits to the hospitals and paying for parking in some hospitals can add up quickly. Taking off work and not being able to make up for paid time lost is very frustrating. The cost of medicine because insurance does not cover certain prescriptions can cause lots of stress.

One of the ways I deal with grief is by trying to look at the positives of caregiving. I know this sounds cliché, but I truly do. I am thankful that God gives me strength and the mental capacity to take care of my son. It does get rough sometimes, but God's word reminds me in Psalm 34:18 that He is "close to the brokenhearted". I am also humbled that I have the ability to help someone that can't help themselves. Caregiving reminds me that life is so fragile, and we must show compassion in the midst of our grief. We are in a time where technology keeps us from face-to-face communication that caregiving is, in some ways, a form of intimate communication.

I find myself taking pride in being a caregiver for my son. It allows us to have small, intimate moments with just the two of us. It is during these times that he'll share how he feels about having Type 1 diabetes or who his friend is at school or share something funny he saw on a cartoon. This brings me joy and is gratifying, knowing that through this disease, our bond is strengthening.

Pause & Ponder

Have you experienced grief since diagnosis?

_____

_____

_____

_____

If so, what are some things you find yourself grieving?

_____

_____

_____

_____

In your moment of grief, where do you find your joy?

_____

_____

_____

_____

Finances
The Business Side of Life

"Therefore, do not worry about tomorrow, for tomorrow will worry about its own things." Matthew 6:34

Taria

Money and finances are one of, if not, the most taboo topics amongst people. Not many people want to talk about what finances look like for their family. One of the many things I love about social media is how people can connect anonymously on a more intimate level. You can find so many Instagram or Facebook accounts where people discuss their finances, their family budget and their debt-free dreams. We firmly believe with the rising cost of healthcare and prescription drugs, it's important to us to be transparent about money and finances. When you are faced with an unexpected diagnosis, in a perfect world, you'd have months and months of savings at your disposal, but we know that is not the case for many of us. When Trace was diagnosed with Type 1, it definitely wasn't the case for us. As previously discussed, I was a SAHM, we were making ends meet but we didn't have a lot of extra money at our disposal. Then add in his diagnosis. After 3 days in the hospital, the doctor wrote Trace a prescription for 3 weeks-worth of needles, insulin, and test strips. When Tyrece got to the pharmacy counter to check out, the bill was over $300 for a few weeks of supplies! This was one of the biggest reality checks as to what we were in store for or what we could expect of our new lives. I immediately began to calculate how much keeping Trace alive was going to cost us each month and in total each year, and this was before we began thinking about the cost of the devices such as an insulin pump and CGM.

I am the planner and budgeter/CFO of our family, our activities and finances. Before Trace was born, we were a two-income family. I had always wanted to stay home with my children "in a perfect world" but I never allowed myself to believe it would happen. I always thought we'd have to be a two-income family. I mean, let's face it, at the time, I had two college degrees that I would be paying on for the rest of my life, I definitely wouldn't be a SAHM anytime soon. We had a mortgage, car payments and credit card debt. As long as we were able to pay a little more than the minimum on our credit cards and had a small savings, I believed we were good. As I mentioned before, we weren't rich by any means but we did have the means to do the things we wanted to do.... eating out, date nights, many trips to Target for needs AND wants etc.

When Trace was born and it was decided I would be staying home, we didn't have a specific timeframe for if and when I would return to work. We just decided to "play it by ear" but knew we would have to get creative with our budget and begin to cut back. At the time, cutting back meant we'd have more meals at home, eat out less, I would limit my Target runs and we would begin to think about getting out of debt. As for healthcare and medical costs, we were okay in that area as well. Our biggest medical bills were the ones that came during pregnancy and after having our kids. We were able to make payments on some of the delivery costs while pregnant and after we took advantage of no interest payments for the remainder of our hospital balances.... cool! I'd planned to keep as much as possible in savings and pay the bills in full whenever feasible. Our only prescriptions were asthma meds for Tate and his Epi pen. Everything was affordable, manageable and in budget. Each year when open enrollment came around, prescriptions for Tate were the only things we had to consider when choosing insurance plans.

After diagnosis, finances and insurance plans were also aspects of our lives that changed. Along with the daily struggle of managing this disease, comes the financial struggle and burden many families face each month. A family like ours, with insurance, can spend hundreds to thousands of dollars per month for the insulin and supplies (needles, lancet devices and lancets, blood sugar meters, test strips etc.) their child needs to survive. If you've ever gone to the doctor or had to stay in the hospital you know medical care is EXPENSIVE!

No matter how good your insurance is, if you have a chronically ill child you know how important finances become and staying on top of never-ending bills. Enter the decision for me to return to work as a school counselor. The bills and medical expenses had begun to weigh too heavily on us, our debt-free dream had been placed on hold. This was probably one of the next biggest decisions Tyrece and I had to make in our marriage. We were at a place in our lives where me staying at home was beneficial for our family and necessary for Trace but our debt had increased and our savings had shrunk.

Trace being diagnosed with Type 1 diabetes impacts every decision we make as a family and it greatly impacts decisions we make in regards to finances and career choices. What opportunities to take or pass up, what salary is acceptable or not, what type of healthcare plan is provided and what prescriptions are covered, how flexible the employer is and the ability to take time off when needed.... are all things that have to be considered.

As I write this chapter, we have gone full-circle and I am now staying home again, while I begin to focus on growing our various business ventures. My most recent counseling position was a grant-funded position. After three years, the grant funds came to an end and we were at another crossroads. We knew with previous experience, the amount of time I had to take off work and with Trace starting Kindergarten, it would be difficult to find a flexible counseling job that would allow me to take time off when needed, oftentimes at the last minute.

We had to weigh our options......

Money or Peace?

Money or Anxiety?

Money or Health?

Money or Trace's safety?

Peace, less anxiety, health and safety won! With a budget plan, of course! I can truly say God blessed us to be in a better position this time around, we are more prepared for medical costs, we've been able to save, we are still on a debt-free journey and closer than ever to being (credit card) debt-free. We have a peace that only He can give us in regards to money.

THAT WILL BE ALL.

John 14: 1
Let not your heart be
troubled, you believe
in God, believe also
in me.

Tyrece

I am so thankful for my wife! I can honestly say I have not worried nor am I concerned knowing she is managing our finances. Although I joke about her long trips to Target and ask "did you spend all of our money?" I know she is going to make sure she looks for deals and coupons and that our family has everything we need. Through everything we've gone through, she supports each and every career decision I make. These decisions don't come easy. Insurance is always will be at the forefront of every decision. With salary being a very close second. As I previously shared, one of my major fears is not being able to afford insulin or other diabetes supplies for Trace. We've been in a position where the bills were long and money was short, however, putting any amount aside for upcoming expenses helps relieve that stress. Even if the amount saved is only $50 for a particular month, when we get a bill for $100, knowing we have something in savings helps us both breathe better. I am happy that early on, we made this a priority in our budget.

In the remainder of this chapter, we have provided you with some resources, tips and strategies that help us and we hope you find helpful, especially if you are responsible for the finances in your household or in your role as primary caregiver.

Finance Tips and Tidbits

You WILL have to make more calls on your child's behalf than you can imagine!

You WILL have more paperwork than you probably ever had before!

Organization will be a must. It looks different for each of us, but a system will save your sanity.

Consider starting a binder, notebook or bin specifically for medical information, important papers, bills etc.

Budget medical bills, prescription costs, doctors' visits etc.:

1. Start off with keeping a notebook or list of monthly costs for each of these items. Take a look at your bank and credit card statements to get an idea of what is spent on a monthly basis.
2. Use this information to begin forming your medical budget. If you are not able to set aside the exact amount each month, set aside what you can. Many of the finance experts will say cut this and that from your budget in order to save but we personally know when managing a chronic illness some things can't be cut from one month to the other. So, save what you can!
3. As you get better each month with budgeting and (possibly) cutting things from your budget, your medical savings will begin to increase, little by little.
4. If you receive a year-end bonus from work or if you're fortunate enough to receive a tax refund, make a goal of putting most if not all, of that lump sum in your medical savings fund.
5. Budgeting and planning are a form of self-care! Over time, it can reduce stress.

MONTHLY BUDGET TRACKING SAMPLE

Month:	Actual	Forcasted	Monthly Savings Goal
Total			

YEARLY BUDGET TRACKING SAMPLE

	Office Visits	Prescriptions	Medical Supplies	Equipment	Other
JAN					
FEB					
MAR					
APR					
MAY					
JUNE					
JULY					
AUG					
SEPT					
OCT					
NOV					
DEC					
Total Spent					
Yearly Savings Goal					

· Keep a list of medical providers:

Along with a new diagnosis, comes a new set of doctors and/or specialists. If your kids are anything like ours, we have several doctors and specialists to keep track of; a Pediatrician, an Endocrinologist, an ENT (ear, nose & throat), Asthma and Allergy specialist and a Neurologist! Keeping up with each of these providers could be a nightmare if I didn't take the time to organize their information. It is also important because, as we settle into our caregiver roles, there is usually one spouse or relative that knows more information than the other. Because of this, it is important to have this information handy just in case another individual needs access to the information.

Begin keeping a list of each medical provider's information.

Medical Contact List

Child:

Provider's Name:

Provider's Specialty:

Phone:

Address:

Hours:

Visit Schedule:

Visit Notes:

Questions to Ask:

School/Work Info

As with medical providers, it is also important to keep information organized for school and/or work. Along with diagnosis or illness management, also comes numerous meetings at the school to ensure your child gets the health and educational services he/she requires.

School Contact List

Teacher

Name: _____

Phone: _____

Email: _____

School Nurse

Name: _____

Phone: _____

Email: _____

504 Coordinator

Name: _____

Phone: _____

Email: _____

Other

Name: _____

Phone: _____

Email: _____

Other

Name: _____

Phone: _____

Email: _____

Advocate!

Don't stop
advocating
for yourself
& your child!

What's been a major cost in your caregiver journey?

_____

_____

_____

_____

How do you cope with the added financial expenses?

_____

_____

_____

_____

What relieves stress for you as it relates to financial stress?

_____

_____

_____

_____

Faith

faith

/fāTH/

noun

complete trust or confidence in someone or something for which there
is no proof

**"Now faith is the substance of things hoped for, the evidence of
things not seen" Hebrews 11: 1**

Taria

Faith is not believing everything will be perfect but it's believing no
matter what, good or bad, God is in control and God will see you
through because His plan is perfect. But is faith hard? Absolutely YES!
Because we are human and seeing things through our emotions and
experiences, it is sometimes hard to see things through our faith lens.
On those hard days and nights, it's hard to say "it is well" and trust

what's going on in our circumstances.

When Trace was first diagnosed (and still) I wrestled with the why's...

why him?

why us?

why this?

why, why, why!???

But God kept bringing to my mind "what if Trace needs this diagnosis to know who God is in his life?" Would I ask why? Would I want it taken away? And to be honest, my answer to these questions are different every time. I sometimes feel okay and say "yes Lord, if this is what Trace needs to know you then I trust your plan" and other days my response is "but Lord, you can do anything, you hold all power, can't you allow Trace to know you and trust you in his life in another way?" Or "there are so many people in this world without Type 1 diabetes trusting and living for God, Trace could be one of them" Or this is the best one "heal Trace and he'll really know who you are and who healed him!" I have to laugh at my own thoughts sometimes! But that's how my human mind rationalizes and copes with our circumstances.

Before Trace's diagnosis (I feel like I say this a lot!) I had faith and I accepted Jesus Christ as my savior as a middle school child. Throughout my young and adult life, I believed He would make things good and right in my life. But the faith I've experienced since being married, having kids, Tate's diagnosis of asthma and then Trace's diagnosis of Type 1 has grown tremendously. There's something about being responsible for other human beings and their lives with no manual, no instructions. The Word of God will show you how little you know and how much you need to depend on a greater strength than your own. That's how I feel about faith. Let's be truthful, we're never in control of our own lives but when we're young or single and only responsible for ourselves, we believe we are, at least I did.

But when your ideology of what you think your life will be comes head-to-head with reality, you start to realize you can't do any of this on your own. That's where faith comes in. With Trace's life and Type 1 diabetes, I know there is nothing I can control. I'm often asked "is Trace's diabetes stable or controlled?" And I have to laugh and think to myself "yep, for the next five minutes!" We were taught how to test blood sugar, how to count carbs, how to factor in exercise or play or sickness or anything else that may affect Trace's blood sugar.....we were taught to believe we could control his diabetes. Just give insulin for the carbs he's eating and he'll be fine! Just give juice or another fast-acting carb for his low blood sugar and he'll be fine! Ha!

We need faith to get through each and every day, each and every night, each and every low blood sugar, each and every high blood sugar, each and every sickness...........Faith is the main source of our strength and support.

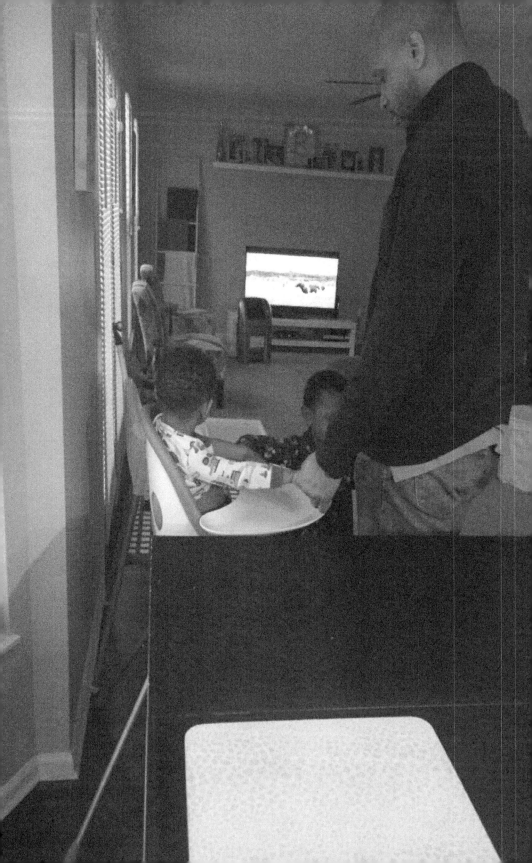

Tyrece

King David in Psalms 121: 1, asks the question, "where does my help come from?" Then he answers his own question by saying, "my help comes from the Lord, which made heaven and earth." This scripture has strengthened my faith over the years but especially with the diagnosis of my son. When I find myself tired from nights of battling high or low blood sugars, I know that my help comes from the Lord. He gives me strength to stay awake. He also shows us favor when Taria and I are too tired to get up in the middle of the night.

I remember one night, we were doing our normal routine of putting the kids to bed. I showered both boys while Taria picked out their clothes for the next day. I helped the boys get their pajamas on and followed up with a story and a scripture verse. I checked Trace's blood sugar, as we do every night before bed, to make sure his blood sugar is not too low or too high. If Trace's blood sugar is high, I will give him insulin to bring his blood sugar down or if he is low, I will give him some apple juice to raise it to a comfortable level.

On this particular night, his blood sugar was in perfect range, it was around 125mg! The CGM also matched the blood sugar reading on the meter and it showed that his blood sugar was steady. In our minds, this means we may have a night of decent sleep, Lord knows we need it!

That night we were both very tired. We set our alarms to 2am for Trace's middle of the night blood sugar check. Because we were so tired, we didn't hear our alarms and we didn't hear his monitor alerting us that Trace had went low. When I woke up the next morning and saw that I missed the alerts and notifications from my phone and didn't hear my alarm clock, I became frantic and had guilt. When I opened my CGM app I saw the graph showing the low blood sugar but it also showed his blood sugar had risen back up and was holding steady at around 111! I also went to his room and did a blood prick sample and it read 115! Science would say that my son experienced what is called

"Dawn Phenomenon" that can occur between the hours of 2am-8am. This is when the body produces hormones that results in a raise in blood sugar. Dawn phenomenon can sometimes be dangerous and cause life threatening high blood sugar.

But we choose to believe God and science, and that morning God reminded me that there is no question of where my help comes from. God has a way to show Himself to let you know that He is there with you in the midst of a storm. We were so tired that night but God allowed us to get our rest. As I reflected on Psalm 121:1, David also says in verse 3, "God does not slumber or sleep." While we were asleep and extremely tired, we know God was actively protecting Trace.

Pause & Ponder

Do you wrestle with asking yourself "why" as you go through this journey?

_____

_____

_____

_____

How would you describe your faith?

_____

_____

_____

_____

Has your faith shifted since diagnosis? If so, in what way?

_____

_____

_____

_____

Balance and Self-Care

"Come to Me, all you who labor and are heavy laden, and I will give you rest." Matthew 11:28

Taria

Is there really such a thing as balance? Self-care?

Seriously, how do you balance the 24-hour care of another human being while taking care of your own personal needs/wants?

As a Type 1 parent, I often feel as if I have to be a mathematician, doctor, nurse, dietician and parent all at once. At any given moment of any day, I am counting carbs, calculating the amount of insulin I think Trace should have based on what he's eaten or what activity he's participated in. I also do a lot of research and read articles on how certain carbs or fat are digested in the body. Then we are triaging any and every issue that comes up in between. Now, add on wife, daughter, sister, friend, employee, business owner etc., and all of these roles and responsibilities can make you TIRED!!!! Chronic illness interrupts everything! Sleep, fun, family time, vacation, school, summer camp, work, date night, birthday parties.....freakin LIFE!!!! But what do you do??! Keeping your child alive is MOST important!!!

Mental health is important under any circumstances. However, with parenting and managing the illness of a chronically sick child, it becomes that much more important. When you are managing an illness and taking care of another human being, it is so easy and common to get lost in those responsibilities. So much so that it becomes who you are, it becomes your identity and sadly, things that previously made you happy or fulfilled get thrown to the wayside.

"If I can't (or wouldn't) say it to someone else in the same situation, don't say it to myself."

This has become my new mantra after going to therapy. My therapist said this statement to me after I kept talking about how I should be dealing with my son's diagnosis better and how I should not still be grieving. Wow!!! That was my exact thought when she said that to me. She was so right! As a school counselor, a friend, a wife, a daughter etc., I would never tell someone to get over their grief. Positive self-talk is a necessary form of self-care that we all must adopt. Positive self-talk is so important and it's ok to not be ok.
Find your community, find your tribe, find your group that understands what you're going through, people in the trench of life, and lean on them. Every month or so, I have a group of girlfriends that will get together for a ladies' night and that's my time to get away for a while.

And one of my absolute favorite things to do is taking a long walk around Target! My therapist recommended that while on these walks around Target, if Trace is with Tyrece or someone else I trust, silence the alarms to truly allow myself some peace, and this has been a lifesaver!

63

Advocate

Support system

"In my distress I called upon the LORD, and cried out to my God; He heard my voice from His temple, And my cry entered His ears."
II Samuel 22:7 NKJV

Strength

Gratitude

Tyrece

Self-care has been very vital for me. It should be vital for anyone that is a caregiver. I never knew or thought that being able to just have 30 minutes of alone time would be so rare and much needed. Being able to sit still and let your body and mind relax is something I took for granted. I've always been a person that likes to be outdoors doing chores; cutting grass has been one of my favorites things to do. I despise when winter comes around and I am not able to go out and cut grass.

Those couple of hours cutting grass help me to relax my mind. Even in the dog days of summer, it is still very relaxing to me. I've realized that it's not that I am away from my son's illness for a couple of hours that gives me joy but rather me being able to control something, physically, that I am not able to control in my son's illness that gives me satisfaction. I can control the length of the grass, the direction of the cut and know that it will last a week or so. I know it sounds a little crazy, but being able to control or tame something after managing Trace's diabetes is like a victory for me. Being outdoors also allows me time to put on my Air Pods, listen to music and clear my mind.

I also love to do one of America's pastimes…grill! Grilling for me has gone from a like to something I am passionate about. I thought this passion was because I am getting older and that's what older men do. Just the aroma from the grill is relaxing to me but most of all I love being able to control the fire and temperature of my grill. It's mind blowing to me that I take gratification in taming the fire. The fire, to me, is like Type 1 with raging blood sugar going up and down through the day. Even though we have insulin and fast-acting carbs to "control" my son's blood sugar, it can still get chaotic and I can't turn the illness off. If the fire on my grill gets out of hand (which rarely happens) I can always put the fire out and start all over.

Self-Care can look different for everyone, here are some things

you can do for self-care:

Get lost in a good book

Get lost in a good movie or tv series

Netflix and chill with yourself

Start a new hobby or get back into an old one

Allow yourself an hour where you are not responsible for your child, grandchild, etc.

Don't get your coffee to-go from your favorite coffee shop

Plan a girls or guys night with friends you haven't connected with in awhile

Start a new hobby or get back into an old one

Take a nap

Exercise or take a walk

Book a spa/massage/mani/pedi day

Journaling

Planning

Read your bible

Get a haircut or go to the salon

Take a relaxing bath or long shower

Treat yourself to your favorite treat (ice cream, milkshake, cupcake, cheese fries (yum!) etc.).

What does self-care look like for you?

_____

_____

_____

Make a list of things you can do for self-care.

_____

_____

_____

How are you taking time out for yourself?

_____

_____

_____

What do you need to help you prioritize self-care?

_____

_____

_____

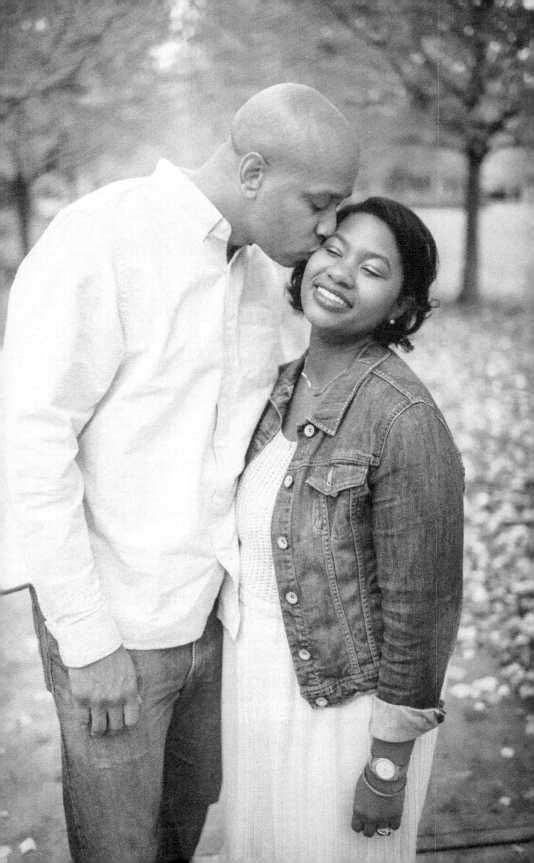

Relationship Care

"Love.....bears all things, believes all things, hopes all things, endures all things." I Corinthians 13:7

T aria

Tyrece and I met in middle school, 6th grade to be exact. We lived one street over from each other until my family moved and I attended a different high school. With that being said, our story isn't a love at first sight story or one where we were middle school loves, not at all. We were friends but that's it, nothing more. Tyrece will say he had a crush on me but that's something I never knew growing up. Fast forward to adult life, our paths crossed a few times but nothing more than a hello and good-bye. In August of 2006, we happened to both be at the same club (gasp!) with friends. He came over to say hello and asked for my phone number. A few days later we went on a lunch date, then another date and before long we were seeing each other regularly and now here we are. We dated for about ten months before becoming an exclusive couple.

During our courtship, like many couples, we focused on getting to know one another; learning about each other's goals and vision for our futures, what trips we would like to take, how many kids we can see ourselves with…you know, all the questions to determine if we were "the one" for one another.

I won't lie, I miss those carefree dating days sometimes. Late dinners, breakfast dates, seeing the latest movie and talking on the phone for hours (uninterrupted!!). As a married couple with kids, one with Type 1 diabetes and the other with Asthma and allergies, it is sometimes difficult to maintain that connection and date like we once did. It gets difficult when you have a child with a special, medical need to find someone to babysit, someone you trust and someone that can handle anything that may arise until you return.

If you're like us, you have to get creative with self-care and relationship care.

Take turns caring for your child, take turns on who gets up at night. We made the huge mistake of not doing this when Trace was first diagnosed and throughout the first year. One reason being that I was not working at the time and Tyrece was. I think we both, unspoken, decided it was necessary for him to get his sleep. That was so wrong on both our parts! To this day, I believe I am still feeling the effects of lack of sleep. Lack of sleep doesn't help with anxiety, migraines, irritability etc. And to this day, I suffer from "alarm fatigue" because it is so hard for me to hear the alerts from Trace's continuous glucose monitor at night.

Alarm fatigue is a term most commonly used for medical professions, particularly nurses. According to the American Association of Critical Care Nurses, it is defined as "desensitization to alarms and missed alarms as a result of constant exposure to said alarms and beeps." Due to an overwhelming number of medical machines equipped with alarms and the number of parents and caregivers responsible for such equipment at home, alarm fatigue is being discussed as an issue for not only medical professionals but also caregivers.

If you're lacking babysitters or other resources for care of your child, think of things that can be done at home. Tyrece and I have had wine and cheese night or movie night when our boys go to bed. We often have to wait for the latest movie to become available for rent on our favorite streaming service rather than going to the movie when they are released. We also do some things separately, and that works for us. If one of our friends are having a birthday party, we decide which of us can go so that at least one of us has an opportunity to get out of the house and have some fun. We don't have a special formula on deciding who gets to attend what event, we just base it on who feels like attending, who seems to need to get out of the house or who's friend it is.

Tyrece

I remember the days of going on dates with my wife and not having a care in the world when it came to finding a babysitter. We would try different restaurants and go see the latest movies. The only thing we had to worry about before Trace's diagnosis was making sure whoever was babysitting our boys knew about Tate's asthma and inhaler, just in case he experienced difficulty breathing, and that they remembered what foods he could and could not eat. We thought back then it was rough making sure people understood the directions on taking care of a kid with asthma and food allergies, boy were we wrong!

Date nights, romance and intimacy are different for us now. Because of Type 1 and the many things that play a role in caring for Trace, we must train family members and friends on all things Type 1 anytime we want to do something without the kids. This has made us get creative with dating, dates now consist of putting the boys to bed, sometimes early, to get a couple of hours of alone time. We've done things like making pizza together, having wine and cheese while listening to music and of course watching a movie. We do not take these moments for granted. These date nights are crucial for our marriage. Sometimes we can get so caught up in taking care of our son that we forget about the bond my wife and I have that started our family. These date nights are us saying we need each other. Romance has taken on a new and different meaning for me.

Romance has been associated with buying flowers, candy and even writing love letters. Romance now is letting my wife sleep a couple hours so that she is well rested for the day, offering her a night at a hotel to get away and relax, or telling her to go to her favorite place to just walk around for a few hours. Romance is showing my wife that we are in this together. The actions of me being there for her are more romantic than any flower or written letter

At-home Date Night Ideas

Wine and cheese night

Movie night

Make a fancy dinner together

20 questions (a way to reconnect)

Wine and canvas painting at home

Game night

Listen to music but each of you take turns playing DJ

5 Ways to (Re)connect

Love Notes

Tyrece and I have a notebook that we dedicated to writing each other notes back and forth, both good and not so good thoughts, as a way to connect. We can admit that it's hard to keep up with and sometimes we forget but making it a priority is always our goal.

Proud, Pleased (thankful) and Prayer

This is where you each write on a sticky note or piece of paper something you are proud of, something you are pleased about or thankful for and something you want the other person to pray for you about. This allows each of us a glimpse into what our partner is thinking or what is on their mind and is ultimately a way to connect.

Date Night Jar

Keep a jar of date night ideas, both at-home and away from home ideas. When a babysitting opportunity arises, pick from the jar to minimize the time it may take to decide what to do with your free time. And the nights when you don't have a babysitter, pick from the at-home ideas to maximize your alone time.

What I need from you

Using post-it notes or notecards, each person writes what they need from the other person. This can be done daily, weekly, monthly….however often. The key will then be to discuss with one another. This small exercise allows each person to communicate what he/she needs from the other person and can eliminate miscommunication and assumptions.

Goal Planning

Grab some notebooks and take some time to goal plan with one another. What are some things each of you want to accomplish individually and as a couple in the next 1 year, 2 years, 5 years, 10 years etc. Goal planning allows you to take a glimpse inside the mind of the other and have some things to look forward to, together!

Get a second opinion

Go to marriage counseling, if needed! Whether it's with your pastor or a licensed therapist, if your marriage seems to need an outside ear or perspective, don't hesitate to make the appointment.

What ways do you stay connected to friends and family?

_____

_____

_____

_____

_____

_____

_____

Brainstorm and list additional ways you can reconnect to your spouse or significant other.

_____

_____

_____

_____

_____

_____

_____

_____

Hope and Encouragement

Not that I speak in regard to need, for I have learned in whatever state I am, to be content:"
Philippians 4:11

Do not weep as if we have no hope........

Taria

Have you ever HOPED so much and so hard for something that it hurts, like literally hurts? Hoping for a cure, hoping for complete healing, hoping for life to be "normal" again, hoping for a good day, week or month, hoping for that miracle that you know God can deliver? This is us, each and every day.

It's HARD taking care of a sick loved one...period!! But you do what has to be done, you cry out to God, you ask "why me?", you even get angry! But then you pray and ask God to give you HIS strength to make it just one more hour, one more day, one more week and so on!!!

There are many days that I am fearful that something bad could happen to Trace, I'm praying at night, I'm praying while he's at school, I'm praying all day! God gives me His strength and I look up and think "wow, we've had a good day, the daycare or school was on top of it today!" and so on and so on. That's finding joy and peace along this journey.

I often feel as if I'm in constant conflict with myself, I have these very extreme thoughts and feelings....Why am I going through this??? But I have hope! Why me?? Why not me?!!! Through every conflicting thought, God continues to assure me that everything is in His hands and He has the final say.

I often find myself thinking "I can't believe this is my life!" It's almost like we're on autopilot so much and so often that I have to wake up from a dream to realize, this is really my (our) life. This is what we're really doing...literally keeping our son alive with every dose of insulin or with every cup of apple juice when his blood sugar is low.

We have to think about and consider the past, present and future in every decision we make for Trace. What he did or ate an hour ago, what he is currently doing and what we plan to do or eat later. EXHAUSTING!! But God knows all these things and more and we have to rest in that each and every day.

Gratitude:

- I am thankful for medical insurance and options!
- I am thankful for Trace's life!
- I am thankful for my husband to share this journey with!

Do I trust God with Trace and his life? Absolutely YES!

God is sovereign over everything, be guided by thankfulness and trust NOT fear.

Don't be afraid to celebrate the successes big and not so big. We find ways to find joy in the journey we are on. In the diabetes community, there is a tern, diaversary. It is the anniversary of one's Type 1 diabetes diagnosis. Some people choose to not celebrate this day, which is understandable, but we choose to celebrate each year.

We celebrate Trace's diaversary because Trace is still here, living and breathing with us! Type 1 diabetes and a blood sugar of 1,000 could have taken our son BUT God saw fit to bless us! To us, this is an instance of finding joy in sorrow, the pain and the bad days. I mourn the life we used to have before Type 1 entered our lives but I thank God every day that Trace still has life to live!!

Isn't it amazing to know that The God that knew us before we were born, The God that formed us in our mothers' wombs knows all about EVERYTHING we're going through, every emotion, every anxiety, every thought! He knew this storm, test or trial was coming and He knows what we need to get through it.

And one day, you'll look up and you're doing so much better, you're more relaxed, less stressed, you're breathing more, you're experiencing less anxiety. And you'll feel like "I got this!" "I can do this!"

And life will throw you more curve balls.... but because of what you've been through and how God has carried you, you know you will make it!

And when you come to that next hard time, that next trial (because it is coming), you'll be able to remember back on how far you've come, how God has kept you, how He has worked things out for you and you will have peace and calmness.

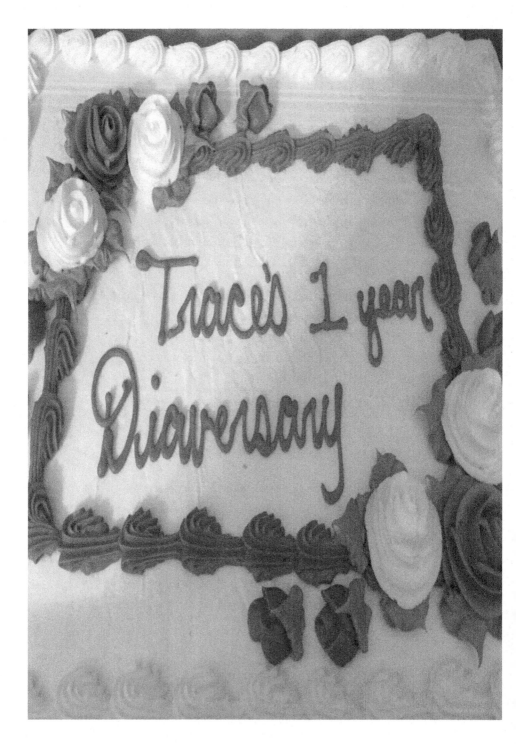

With mixed emotions, TRUST GOD!

Tyrece

There is one passage of scripture that is always on my mind and that I cling on to that gives me hope for our situation. 1 Peter 4:12-13 "Beloved, do not think it strange concerning the fiery trial which is to try you, as though some strange thing happened to you; but rejoice to the extent that you partake of Christ's suffering, that when His glory is revealed, you may also be glad with exceeding joy."

I remember when I was a teenager and a preacher named Paul Davis preached this passage. Never did I think that in a million years this scripture would become real in our lives. We were a young family that did not have a care in the world and then Boom! We were faced with a fiery trial! Like anyone that faces a trial, there are always the questions why me? Why us? And why now? This is a trial that seems to never end.

Trace's illness has certainly been a struggle for us emotionally and physically. I see this trial as an opportunity for us to grow spiritually because we trust that God will bring His purpose through our fiery trial. Sometimes these trials are given to us to show us how much we need God. We can sometimes get too complacent with our relationship with God and become independent from Him. We have to remember that He is our source of strength and refuge when going through our trials.

My hope is that God is revealed through our journey. I hope that anyone that is going through a trial is encouraged to trust God and that He is a present help. My wife and I have not arrived and do not have all the answers to why we go through different circumstances but we are encouraged that He is working through our family's journey to encourage others to trust Him.

What does joy look like for you?

_____

_____

_____

_____

What are some things you would tell someone in your shoes to encourage them?

_____

_____

_____

_____

Use those things to, now, write a letter of encouragement to yourself.

_____

_____

_____

_____

_____

_____

Asking GOD for BIG things!

"Lord my God, I called you for help, and you healed me."

Psalms 30:2

"Not that I speak in regard to need, for I have learned in whatever state I am, to be content:"

Philippians 4:11 NKJV

"In my distress I called upon the LORD, And cried out to my God; He heard my voice from His temple, And my cry entered His ears."

II Samuel 22:7 NKJV

"Give your burdens to The Lord"

Psalms 55:22

"Cast all your care (anxiety) on Him because He cares for you (me)"

 1 Peter 5:7

"The Lord is my (our) strength and my (our) shield, in Him my (our) heart trusts, and I (we) are helped; my heart exults and with my song I give him thanks."

Psalms 28:7

Reflections and Notes

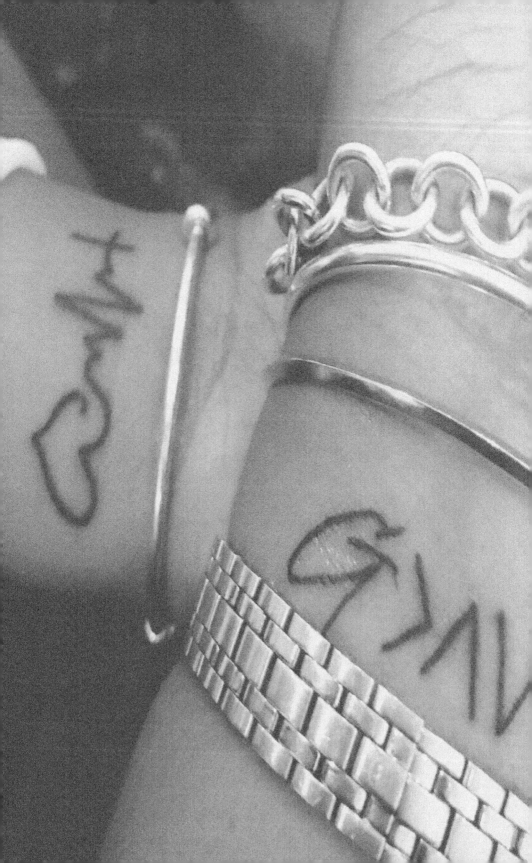

Reflections and Notes

Throughout this book, we have reflected upon our journey. We now invite you to reflect upon your own journey as a caregiver.

Use the space provided to further explore the topics that we discussed in *2am Parenting* and to think about your own story.

_____

_____

_____

_____

_____

_____

_____

_____

_____

_____

_____

_____

_____

_____

_____

_____

_____

_____

_____

_____

Reflections and Notes

Reflections and Notes

Reflections and Notes

Reflections and Notes

Reflections and Notes

Reflections and Notes

Reflections and Notes

Reflections and Notes

Reflections and Notes

Reflections and Notes

Reflections and Notes

Reflections and Notes

Reflections and Notes

Reflections and Notes

Reflections and Notes

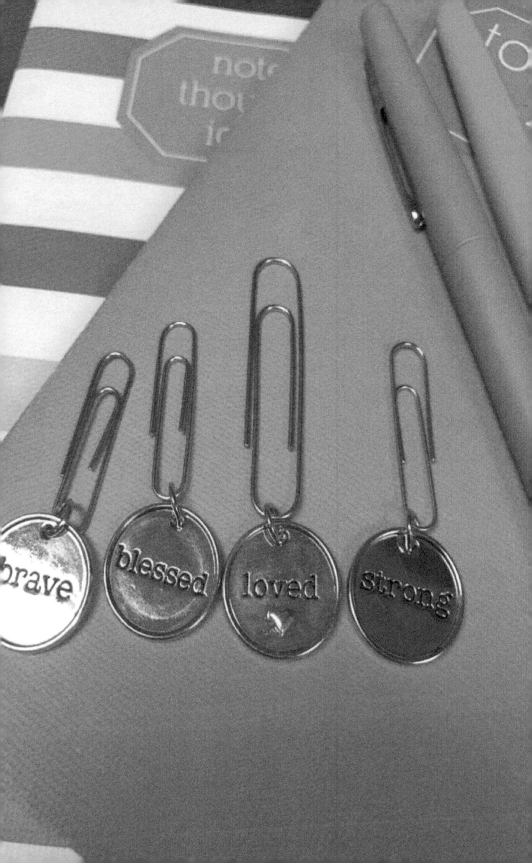

Reflections and Notes

Reflections and Notes

Reflections and Notes

Reflections and Notes

Reflections and Notes

Reflections and Notes

Reflections and Notes

Reflections and Notes

Reflections and Notes

Reflections and Notes

Reflections and Notes

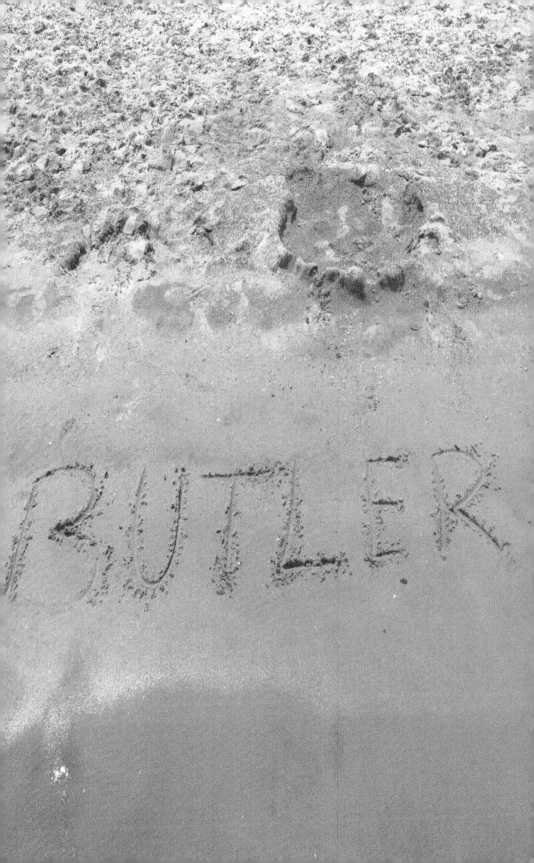

EPILOGUE

As we wrap up this book, Tyrece and I are still on our journey of 2am Parenting. We are committed to parenting our children, nurturing our personal selves and mental health and nurturing our relationship. Writing this book has been very therapeutic for both of us. We hope that this book is what someone needs as they embark on a new journey or continue the journey they've already begun. Our journey still holds ups and downs, highs and lows, good days and bad days and sleepless nights. But we look forward to God continuing to keep us, strengthen us, give us peace and to use our journey to help other families.

We have a nonprofit organization in honor of our son, Trace, The traceBRAVE Foundation. Our nonprofit aims at helping other families with a child or children with Type 1 diabetes with financial and emotional needs and to educate the community about Type 1 diabetes.

www.tracebravefoundation.org

We have also started a t-shirt and apparel company, PrickLife, to bring awareness to Type 1 diabetes in a fun way and to support The traceBRAVE Foundation.

www.pricklife.com

We look forward to what the future holds for us and our family.

Please keep up with us and follow our journey via our website,

www.2amparenting.com
and our social media pages:
Facebook-2amParenting
Instagram-2amparenting

Please reach out to us as you go through your journey and read through the book, we'd love to hear from you!

Thank you for reading and coming along with us!

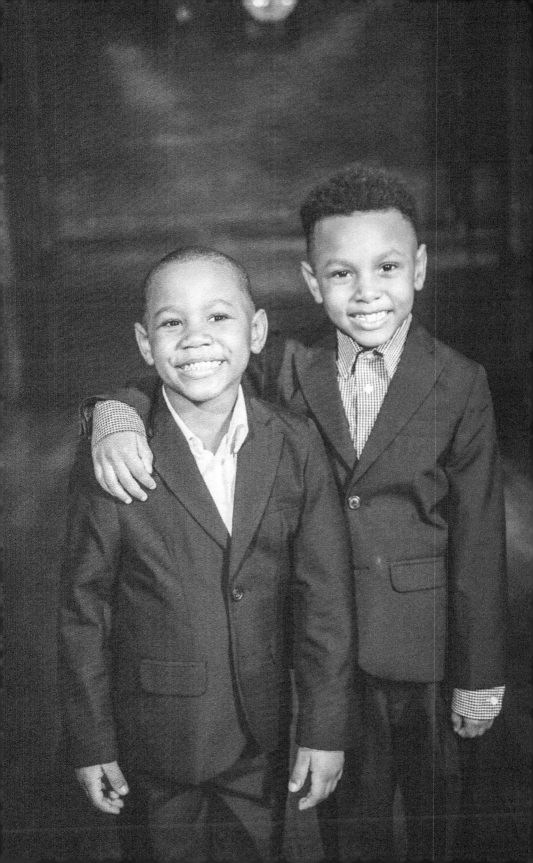

ABOUT THE AUTHORS

Tyrece Butler has a Bachelor's of Arts in Sports Management from the University of Michigan. He serves as the President of The traceBRAVE Foundation, which is a non-profit organization founded to assist families with children diagnosed with Type 1 diabetes. He is also the co-founder of PrickLife, an apparel company bringing awareness to Type 1 diabetes. When not advocating for Type 1 diabetes, Tyrece specializes in sales and leads training workshops on his company's products for each of his clients. Tyrece resides in Indianapolis, Indiana with his wife and two young sons.

Taria Butler, M.S. Ed, M.A. Ed. Psych.
Taria is a licensed School Counselor, formerly serving as a School Counselor for high school aged students. Taria is also the Vice President of The traceBRAVE Foundation, a nonprofit organization that aims to help families with children who have Type 1 diabetes. Lastly, she is the Co-Founder of PrickLife, an apparel company combining fashion and awareness for Type 1 diabetes.

Taria has experience in teaching, coaching and leading small groups in the areas of:
- Type 1 Diabetes Education
- Type 1 Diabetes and School Management
- Goal-setting
- Individual Counseling
- Grief Counseling
- Academic and College/Career Counseling

Taria is also the wife of Tyrece Butler, mother to Tate, age 7 and Trace, age 5, and they reside in Indianapolis, IN.

Made in the USA
Coppell, TX
27 February 2021